OSTEOPOROSIS COOKBOOK

What to Eat and What Not to Eat If You Have Osteoporosis

EVAN BROOKS

Table of Contents

CHAPTER ONE

Foods to eat for osteoporosis

What to Eat and What Not to Eat If You Have Osteoporosis

Osteoporosis prevention necessitates a diet rich in calcium and vitamin D. Avoid these common osteoporosis diet pitfalls for stronger bones. Osteoporosis can be prevented by eating a diet rich in essential nutrients such as calcium, vitamin D, and protein. As an additional bone-health benefit, limiting caffeine and alcohol consumption may be beneficial for older adults.

Salt Is Bad for the Bones in the Osteoporosis Diet

A strong skeleton can be greatly hindered by the presence of salt. Bone mineral loss is greater in postmenopausal women who consume a high-salt diet than in other women of the same age, according to a study.

For example, "the salt content of the typical American diet is a factor in the high level of calcium requirements," says Linda K. Massey of Washington State University in Spokane, an expert in human nutrition.

studies have shown that regular table salt, not just sodium, causes calcium loss and weakens bones over time. This is critical, as salt accounts for the majority of the sodium consumed by the average American.

In addition, we consume far more sodium than we should. According to the 2005 Dietary Guidelines for Americans, a teaspoon of salt contains 2,300 milligrams of sodium per day. However, the average American consumes 4,000 milligrams of the supplement daily.

your body excretes 40 milligrams of calcium for every 2,300 milligrams of sodium you consume.

Calcium and vitamin D supplementation helps to

counteract the effects of salt on bone density.

For adults ages 18 to 50, the equivalent of three 8-ounce glasses of milk is the amount of calcium they need each day.

• The daily calcium requirement for older adults is 1,200 milligrams, or an additional half-glass of milk.

In terms of vitamin D:

• Until the age of 50, people require 200 IU of vitamin D per day.

• Adults between the ages of 51 and 70 need 400 IU of vitamin D daily.

After the age of 70, seniors require 600 IU of vitamin D per day.

Vitamin D can be found in sunlight, fortified milk, egg yolks, saltwater fish, liver, supplements, and fortified foods.

Salt is the most difficult of the bone-damaging elements to avoid. Many processed foods contain salt, including whole grain breads, cereal, and fast food.

It helps to remove the salt shaker from the table, and to cook without adding salt. However, avoiding processed foods is the best way to get the most out of your money. We consume 75% of our sodium intake from processed foods.

Here are some of the saltiest foods to limit or avoid if you want to learn more about this diet danger. Salt-free products should be your first choice whenever possible.

• Deli turkey and ham, hot dogs, and other processed meats

a variety of quick-service restaurants, such as those that serve fast food

In addition to regular and low-calorie frozen meals, processed foods include

Vegetable and tomato juice concentrates in a regular canned soup or stew

- Breads, cereals, and other baked goods

Salt content can be found on food labels. If you're concerned about bone health, it's likely that the majority of it is made up of salt.

When you go out to eat, look up the sodium content of the dishes you most frequently order on the websites of your favorite restaurants. Choose low-sodium options like grilled fish or chicken, steamed vegetables, baked potato, and salad if your typical meals contain more than

800 mg of sodium. Request that your meal be prepared without salt, too.

Eating plenty of potassium-rich foods like bananas and orange juice can help you lower your salt intake. Calcium loss may be reduced by potassium supplementation.

Diet Danger 2: Some Popular Beverages That Increase Risk for Osteoporosis

Soft drinks and some other carbonated soft drinks contain phosphoric acid, which increases the amount of calcium excreted from your body. In addition, most soft drinks are deficient in calcium. Women who are predisposed to osteoporosis should avoid this combination at all costs.

When calcium intake is low, excess phosphorus promotes calcium loss from the body, Massey explains.

However, many people, particularly women, go through more than one can or glass of soda a day. Soft-drink drinkers may also avoid calcium-rich beverages, such as milk, yogurt-based drinks, and calcium and vitamin D fortified orange juice, because they are concerned about their health.

• Eight ounces of calcium- and vitamin D-fortified orange juice

Orange juice with phosphoric acid-free seltzer or club soda is an option.

CHAPTER TWO

Frozen fruit and fat-free yogurt blended together in a blender or food processor with one medium banana or a cup of frozen fruit

In addition, fat-free milk can be found in a variety of flavors, including plain and chocolate.

Consuming Caffeine May Increase Your Risk of Osteoporosis Diet Danger #3

Caffeine weakens bones by stealing calcium from them.

According to Massey, for every 100 milligrams of caffeine consumed, the body loses about 6 milligrams of calcium.

Even if the loss isn't as great as the loss of salt, it's still a cause for concern. When a woman isn't getting enough calcium in her diet, caffeine can be especially dangerous.

If you limit your caffeine intake to 300 milligrams a day and get enough calcium, you may be able to offset some of the negative effects of caffeine, says Massey.

Coffee is one of the most important sources of caffeine. 320 milligrams can be found in a 16-ounce cup of coffee. Cans of high-caffeine sodas can contain as much as 80 milligrams of caffeine per serving..

Despite the fact that it contains caffeine as well, studies show that drinking tea in the elderly does not harm bone density and may even improve it if milk is added. Tea may contain plant compounds that protect bone, according to researchers.

Ready to give up caffeine? A few pointers:

- Begin by consuming half regular and half decaffeinated brews in order to gradually reduce your caffeine intake.

Do not drink any caffeinated beverages, such as coffee, tea, or soda

When it comes to tea, opt for decaffeinated options, like iced tea or hot tea

Decaf, fat-free latte drinks have an added benefit of providing

450 milligrams of calcium per serving.

Danger 4 of the Osteoporosis Diet: Is Protein a Problem?

According to University of Connecticut nutrition professor and bone researcher Jane Kerstetter, PhD, RD, it is a myth that protein, particularly animal protein, is bad for bones. "Bone is not broken down by protein. Quite the contrary, in fact."

About half of the protein in bones is collagen. Dietary amino acids, the building blocks of body proteins, are essential for bone repair.

Protein is a close second in importance to calcium and vitamin D in protecting bone health, according to Kerstetter.

Most Americans get enough protein, but Kerstetter claims that a lot of older women aren't getting enough and it's causing them to suffer from bone loss.

For men and women over the age of 19, the recommended daily protein intake is 0.8 grams of protein per 2.2 pounds. A

150-pound woman needs 55 grams of protein daily, while a 175-pound man needs 64 grams.

• 22 grams of protein in 3 ounces of drained light tuna

There are about 20 grams of protein in 3 ounces of cooked chicken, turkey, or pork tenderloin.

• 19 grams in 3 ounces of cooked salmon

A serving of fat-free plain yogurt contains 13 grams of fat per 8 ounces.

8 grams of fat-free milk per 8 ounces

6 grams of protein in a medium-sized egg

Diet Danger No. 5: There's a Problem with Soy

Despite the high levels of bone-building protein found in soy products like edamame, tofu, and tempeh, as well as in soy beverages, plant compounds present in soy products may interfere with calcium absorption.

the oxalates in soy can bind calcium and render it inaccessible to the body. When eating too much soy but not enough calcium, Kerstetter warns, problems can occur.

Research on soy is inconclusive. The right kind of soy (with the soy isoflavones genistein and daidzein) protects bone strength, according to some small studies. To be safe, make sure to consume plenty of calcium, primarily in the form of dairy products or supplements.

Calcium-fortified soy products may give consumers a false sense of security. [page needed] It was discovered that even after vigorous shaking, a significant amount of calcium in soy and other calcium-fortified beverages settled to the bottom of the container and could not be redistributed throughout the beverage.

Even so, calcium-fortified tofu and other fortified soy products are a good source of bone-building nutrients and a welcome addition to a healthy diet. Make sure you get at least 1,000 milligrams of calcium a day if you eat a lot of soy.

Osteoporosis Diet: The Ultimate Guide

Osteoporosis is difficult to perceive because of the inability to feel the condition, according to Kerstetter. "However, your daily diet is extremely important. It's dangerous in the long run to have a string of bad eating days."

CHAPTER THREE

Foods high in fresh and minimally processed whole grains, fruits and vegetables are the safest bet for a healthy diet. Avoid caffeine and carbonated drinks, and make sure you're getting enough calcium and vitamin D from your diet.

Bone health is influenced by a person's diet.

Because of the constant breakdown and rebuilding that occurs as part of normal bone metabolism, bone does not remain static throughout life.

Involvement of Trusted Source, Osteoblasts and Osteoclasts The process of resorption occurs when osteoblasts create new bone and osteoclasts decompose old bone.

Bone density, strength, and brittleness can all decrease if bone metabolism is out of whack. Osteoporosis or low bone mass may be diagnosed as a result.

A number of variables come into play.

Bone loss can occur as a result of aging, menopause, and some medications.

Osteoporosis risk can be reduced by consuming essential nutrients for bone health.

People who want strong bones should eat a diet rich in the nutrients and foods listed below:

Calcium

calcium deficiency throughout life has been linked to low bone mass and high fracture rates by the National Institute of Arthritis and Musculoskeletal and Skin Diseases.

For women, 1,200 milligrams (mg) of calcium a day is required, while men require 1,000 mg.

Dairy and soy products, fish with bones, and leafy green vegetables can all help people get the calcium they need in their diets.

The following is a list of foods that contain a significant amount of calcium:

350 mg calcium in each packet of fortified oatmeal.

• canned sardines with edible bones, 3 oz: 324 mg calcium

Calcium content per serving: 306 mg in 1.5 ounces of shredded cheddar cheese.

1 cup nonfat milk contains 302 mg of calcium.

The calcium content of 0.5 cups of firm tofu with calcium is 204 mg per serving

• 6 oz of orange juice, calcium-enriched: 200–260 mg calcium

(142mg calcium per cup of baked beans)

Vitamin D is essential for a healthy immune system.

Vitamin D is required for the body to absorb calcium, and a deficiency in vitamin D may lead to bone and skeletal system weakness.

Vitamin D is recommended for people ages 20 to 70, according to the advice of nutritionists.

If you're 70 or older, your dietary intake should be increased to 800 IU per day.

CHAPTER FOUR

In addition to sunlight and food, people can obtain vitamin D. Vitamin D can be found in the following foods:

in addition to the egg yolk

Salmon, trout, mackerel, and tuna are good sources of omega-3 fatty acids.

In addition, beef liver can be found.

• cheese

• mushrooms that have been treated with ultraviolet light by their growers

Added vitamin D to milk, margarine, orange juice and breakfast cereals

Protein

Diverse studies have produced conflicting results regarding the effects of protein on bone health and suggest that it can be both beneficial and detrimental to bone health.

Framingham

OsteoporosisTrusted Source study, however, shows that low protein intake is associated with greater bone loss and hip fractures in older adults.

Bone mineral density appears to improve when adequate protein and calcium intake is combined, according to a new study (BMD).

A diet high in protein and calcium is therefore recommended. The following are examples of protein-rich foods:

• meat

- fish

- eggs

The following are examples of dairy products:

For example: • legumes such as beans

products made from soybeans

- seitan

Pistachios and other tree nuts

Fruits and vegetables are rich in micronutrients and antioxidants.

Higher fruit and vegetable consumption was linked to better bone density and less bone loss in the Framingham Osteoporosis Study.

Bone health benefits from fruit and vegetable consumption include the following.

Vitamin C is an important nutrient for the body.

Vitamin K is an essential nutrient.

- magnesium

- potassium

- folate

- carotenoids

According to a study of Chinese people aged 40–75, those who eat more fruits and vegetables have a lower risk of developing osteoporosis.

Also in 2019, there was a meta-analysis of these studies

People who eat at least one serving of fruits and vegetables each day are less likely to fracture their bones, according to a study published in Trusted Source.

Eating too many of these foods

In addition to a healthy diet, people should be aware of some foods and beverages that can harm bone health.

Salt

Calcium is excreted from the kidneys when the kidneys are overloaded with salt,
This is why people who do not get enough calcium from diets rich in calcium-rich foods should limit their salt intake.

Phytates and oxalates are found in a number of foods.

If you're concerned about calcium absorption, the Bone

Health and Osteoporosis Foundation recommends avoiding certain foods.

Beans, wheat bran, and legumes, as well as spinach and beets, contain oxalates. To reduce these compounds, soak and cook these foods.

Alcohol

For a variety of reasons, experts believe that drinking alcohol can harm bone health.

The body's ability to absorb calcium and vitamin D can be

hindered by excessive drinking of alcohol.

The hormone cortisol, which is elevated by heavy drinking, can break down more bone if it is consumed on a regular basis. As testosterone production declines in men, bone formation may be compromised, while women may experience irregular menstrual cycles. Osteoporosis risk is increased when a woman has irregular menstrual cycles, which lowers her estrogen levels.

In addition, people who are intoxicated are more likely to suffer a fall or break a bone.

Caffeine

A 2021 study found that the kidneys' clearance of calcium was increased by 77% when 800 mg of caffeine was consumed over six hours.

In a previous study, researchers found that people should limit themselves to no more than three cups of coffee a day, especially if they are elderly.

Another source of calcium depletion is the caffeine found in soft drinks like cola, according to the Bone Health and Osteoporosis Foundation.

Summary

Eat a diet rich in nutrients and engage in regular exercise to keep bones strong throughout one's life.

Fruits and vegetables contain a wide range of vitamins, minerals, and antioxidants, including calcium, vitamin D, and protein.

Drinking too much coffee or alcohol is not recommended for people over the age of sixty-five.

Those who do not consume enough calcium may benefit from limiting their intake of alcohol and salt, which can have a positive impact on overall health and well-being.

THE END

www.ingramcontent.com/pod-product-compliance
Lightning Source LLC
Chambersburg PA
CBHW050619160726
48003CB00003B/1245